The Hot Sauce Diet

The Hot Sauce Diet

✦

A journey of behavior modification

Spiro B. Antoniades, M.D.
With illustrations by Ian Jones

iUniverse, Inc.
New York Lincoln Shanghai

The Hot Sauce Diet
A journey of behavior modification

iUniverse books may be ordered through booksellers or by contacting:

iUniverse
2021 Pine Lake Road, Suite 100
Lincoln, NE 68512
www.iuniverse.com
1-800-Authors (1-800-288-4677)

You should not undertake any diet regimen recommended in this book before consulting your personal physician. Neither the author nor the publisher shall be responsible or liable for any loss or damage allegedly arising as a consequence of your use or application of any information or suggestions contained in this book.

ISBN-13: 978-0-595-41187-0 (pbk)
ISBN-13: 978-0-595-85544-5 (ebk)
ISBN-10: 0-595-41187-8 (pbk)
ISBN-10: 0-595-85544-X (ebk)

Printed in the United States of America

Contents

Acknowledgements

I would like to thank Andrew Hayden for his thoughtful editorial efforts and also my wife Christina who has supported me by endlessly editing my manuscript, encouraging my eccentric endeavors, and raising our three children.

1

How to Make a Pig Fly

"Pigs may fly but it's not likely"[1]. The old Scottish proverb rings true, and that's what makes it sweet to defy. On May 7th, 2006 at 6 a.m. I stood in a crowd of 14,911 people to prove the Scottish proverb wrong. I was running in the 2006 Flying Pig Marathon in Cincinnati, Ohio.

The city was named after a virtuous country farmer, Lucius Quintus Cincinnatus, who twice led 5th century Rome to military victory against invaders. The city of Cincinnati later named its marathon in honor of its long history as a meat packing and processing mecca.

For me, it was a day of triumph. I celebrated reaching a higher level. A pig was flying. Wearing nothing but a tank top, shorts and running shoes, my 39-year-old, 5'11" 190-pound frame was bare to the harsh elements. I looked no different than most of the crowd and felt comfortable.

A year ago I was 70 pounds heavier and deeply ashamed of my own body. I was a glutton. Although my life was happy and fulfilled, every time I looked in the mirror I knew my external shape wasn't the real me. It had taken me years of ignoring my health to pack on the pounds, but just one year of serious commitment to undo the damage.

On that day I stood proud to blend in among the thin and robust. A lot of you may think, so what? Some may be thinking; how did you do it?

The short answer is hot sauce. If you want the long answer, keep reading.

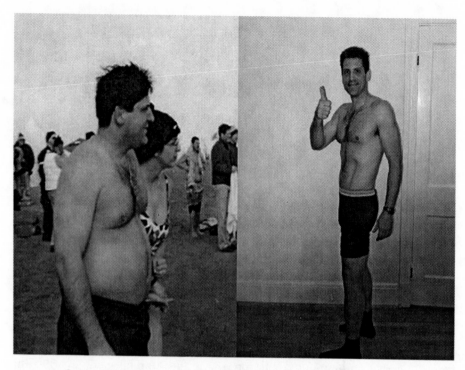

On the left pre-hot sauce diet January 2005 and on the right post-hot sauce diet eleven months later (December 2005).

2

Rock Bottom

My story begins a year prior with the day I reached rock bottom. I was in my doctor's waiting room patiently waiting. Being a doctor myself, I take great pains to display extraordinary patience when waiting for my doctor. This way I can make everyone wait on me without a guilty conscience. I brought plenty to read and was very comfortable and content. Away from my own office, it was a time for me to relax. Slouching in the chair, I comfortably rested the lower edge of the magazine on the crease between my abdomen and chest, just below the nipple line. My belly jetted out of my trunk at a near 90-degree angle. I chuckled at the resourceful use of my distended anatomy. Before long a nurse's aide called my name. Time to see the doctor.

The first order of business was stepping on the scale. What was the point of measuring my weight? First of all, everyone knows that scales are notoriously inaccurate. The one in my bathroom varies by five pounds depending on whether I'm leaning backwards or forwards. Just spreading my gnarly toes to see the weight made me two pounds lighter. Which measurement do you use?

Second, measured weight is a mere snapshot in time. It varies from day to day and during the day. It had no real meaning to me in the last several years. I've lost weight in the past, so I firmly believed I could always do it again. And anyhow, my current bathroom scale never decreases no matter what type of diet I try. I can never believe what the scale reads because it is just way too high.

Third, who cares what I weigh? Why is it the doctor's business to weigh me? I'm married with three children under five years of age. Does anybody really care what I look like? The main reason my wife even looks at me is to make sure she has just enough eye contact so that I can't refuse the latest chore. One of my best friends from residency told me at a meeting I had become an "old fat guy." I somehow rationalized my weight in a delusion of grandeur as a filandering force-field to block the imaginary hordes of lascivious women from noticing me. My family comes first!

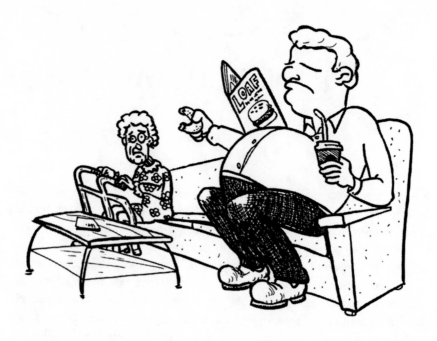

Practical uses for a robust physique while waiting in the doctor's office.

Who was I kidding?

Fourth, what is the point of measuring weight? If you use the actuarial tables for optimal weight, for my height of 5'11" I would have to be a 99 pound weakling! I rationalized my weight with the fact that I could bench press more than 300 pounds, and that the height and weight tables are for pencil-necked geeks, not for weight lifters. (I still considered myself a weightlifter, even if it was only for one to two half-hearted twenty-minute sessions each month).

The nurse's aide didn't even hesitate to start the measurements at 200 pounds. It made an embarrassingly loud CLUNK! I thought the whole office could hear it. How dare she assume I weigh over 200? She gave me the dignity of starting the smaller top weight at 210 and slowly increasing the pounds. The scale didn't budge...210...220...230...240...248! YIKES! My heart sunk. I thought I had lost 5 pounds recently. Maybe the scale was off.

When the nurse's aid wrote 248 on my chart, I was a little resentful. How accurate was the weight? Who cared? It's none of their business! She led me down the hall. I imagine she was probably thinking, "Let's go, Chubs...."

Was I overweight? What should I weigh?

Understanding BMI

The most objective measure of weight is Body Mass Index (BMI)[2]. It is a number that shows body weight adjusted for height. Body Mass Index can be calculated using pounds and inches with this equation:

$$BMI = \frac{\text{Weight in Pounds}}{(\text{Height in inches}) \times (\text{Height in inches})} \times 703$$

For example, I weighed 248 pounds and was 5'11" so my BMI was 34.6.

$$\frac{248 \text{ lbs.}}{(72 \text{ inches}) \times (72 \text{ inches})} \times 703 = 34.6$$

I've listed the BMI ranges below:

BMI below 18.5 = Underweight
BMI 18.5–24.9 = Normal
BMI 25.0–29.9 = Overweight
BMI 30.0 and above = Obese

I had to be 179 pounds, or lose 69 pounds to fall in the normal range!

Is BMI balderdash? The scientific medical literature doesn't think so. A high BMI is without question associated with significantly increased rates of death and disabling disease. If a man's waistline is the same as my former 40-inch waist (for a woman it's 35 inches), there is an *additional independent* risk of heart disease.

But I'm a weightlifter! It's true that BMI doesn't account for muscle mass. But here you must be realistic. Do I need to lift 350 pounds off my chest? Is this a priority in my life? For meathead-mentality reasons in high school and college, strength was a priority. At 38, I could no longer claim it was. I do say this with some remorse.

Now wait a minute! If you insert four-time all-pro Baltimore Raven linebacker Ray Lewis into the equation you get a height of 6'1" and weight of 245 lb., which yields a BMI of 32.3. Does that mean Ray Lewis is obese? No. Not by any stretch of the imagination. The fact is there probably are extraordinarily few people who have Ray Lewis' physique. In a study where BMI was compared to actual fat content in the same patients, BMI was found to be an excellent estimate of adiposity[3] or fat content. In other words, for the vast majority of us the formula works very well to predict fat content. The Ray Lewis example is a fluke.

What's your BMI? Take a break and figure it out, it's important.

The Moment of Truth

Let's go back to my day at the doctor's office. I had progressed to the next waiting area in the small examining room. The walls were covered with children's stickers of planets and rockets for the pediatric population in the office. I sat on the crinkly paper. At the request of the nurse, my shirt was off. When the nurse looked at my extended hairy belly, she hesitated and probably thought about asking me to put my shirt back on. After a second look she turned suddenly and walked out the door. I sat there alone looking at my belly button. It added to the detached surreal experience I was having.

My doctor bolted into the room in a rush and immediately took my blood pressure, which wasn't bad at 125/85. His quick barrage of questions and fast movements were in stark contrast to the slow silent wait that preceded him. He then went over the blood test results that I had taken the week before. My cholesterol was 256 and my glucose was 120. He started rattling off reasons why the numbers were high and he went into some details that I immediately tuned out.

I was in a state of shock. I started rationalizing the cholesterol level. Maybe I ate one too many steaks last week. An elevated glucose level, however, was *not* negotiable in my mind.

Diabetes?

What is Adult Onset Diabetes, otherwise known as Non-insulin Dependent Diabetes Mellitus (NIDDM) or Type II Diabetes Mellitus? As defined by my Stedman's Medical Dictionary[4],

> "…Adult Onset Diabetes is an often mild form of diabetes mellitus of gradual onset, usually in obese individuals over age 35; absolute plasma insulin levels are normal to high, but relatively low in relation to plasma glucose levels…it responds well to dietary regulation and/or oral hypoglycemic agents, but diabetic complications and degenerative changes can develop."

Diabetes is a metabolic disease process where your body cannot break down and use the sugar in your blood stream. The glucose level in the blood increases to abnormally high levels. Your body is starving for sugar while swimming in a sea of it. An abnormally high glucose level in your blood, over time, can destroy blood vessels in the heart, brain and lower extremities. This can lead to heart attacks, strokes, potential loss of limbs and can result in the body being more susceptible to infections.

Diabetes in Action

The thought of diabetes brings me back to one of my formative experiences as a doctor. I think of it whenever I hear the word. I had just graduated from The Johns Hopkins University School of Medicine. I knew almost everything there was to know about medicine, or at least as much as you can cram into four short years. I was in the middle of my first year as a cocksure surgery intern covering the emergency room for the orthopaedic service consultations.

It's been 14 years, but I clearly remember the digits 2626 from the emergency room that would constantly beep on my pager. I think they are tattooed somewhere in my brain. They meant, "I don't care how tired you are, how inexperienced you are, or how little you have slept, just wake up and get down here for some more."

It was the middle of the night and I was still rubbing the sleep out of my eyes when the battleaxe emergency room nurse pointed to the chart on the rack. You may know the type: bitter and mean after years of dueling with nasty doctors and demanding patients in the middle of their own personal emergency. They wear the designer teddy bear scrubs that contrast with their sandpaper personality.

"It's a diabetic foot for you they signed out to me" she muttered as she finished off the last donut in a box left over from the last shift. In other words, she hadn't yet seen the patient, who had probably been sitting neglected and stewing for five hours.

I grabbed the chart and looked at the scrawl for clues. I have always enjoyed being a doctor. When I was thirteen I read the entire works of Arthur Conan Doyle. Sherlock Holmes was my hero. I always imagined myself a sleuth sniffing out the details, cataloging relevant facts and figures in my mind and putting my deductive reasoning skills to the test. In my own mind I was walking the foggy dimly-lit streets of 19th century London with my walking cane and pipe, Dr. Watson at my side.

I had no idea what I was going to see for the first time.

The first order of business was age and sex (45 years and female) and chief complaint of the patient ("I don't feel good"). At this point without having met the patient I would try to make my diagnosis. Although I had only four things to work on I knew it must be a diabetic patient with a foot infection. Diabetics are prone to infections, and the infection was making her feel ill. I looked further at the chart to see the vital signs and labs. She had a slight fever of 101.5, elevated heart rate of 110 beats per minute and a slightly elevated respiratory rate of 15 breaths per minute. Her labs revealed an elevated white blood cell count of 13,000 and an elevated glucose level of 300. All of these facts were consistent with an infection. The infection was probably stressing her diabetic condition and her glucose levels were possibly about to spiral out of control. Next came the exam.

The patient was sitting in a chair in the corner of the room in a tattered blue terrycloth bathrobe with matching slippers. Her hair was disheveled and she smelled of cigarette smoke, alcohol and blood. I will forever associate the emergency room with this cocktale of odors. Her face was wrinkled and worn and she appeared older than her chronologic age. She was quietly crying. One of her slippers was slightly stained at the front with what appeared to be dried blood. An intravenous line was in her arm dripping antibiotics from a bag that hung from the ceiling. Immediately these facts gave me more insight. Anyone who suffers from diabetes who smokes and drinks alcohol is really asking for trouble. She was possibly in denial of her disease and probably addicted to alcohol and cigarettes.

I asked her what brought her to the emergency room and she said, "I just haven't felt well the last couple of days." I asked her if her sugar was under control and she said no.

At that point it was time to go where the money was so I asked her to remove her slipper to look at her foot. She slowly lifted her foot off the ground and removed her slipper without once looking down at her own foot.

I couldn't believe what I saw. The slipper was full of small pieces of colored broken glass, I assumed from a beer bottle. The sole of the slipper was covered with dry blood. Her foot was swollen to twice the size of the opposite side and was beet red up to the ankle. The bloodied sole of her foot was dotted with different-sized pieces of glass, some buried deep in the skin, others halfway through. I reflexively grimaced.

She looked at me and said, "What's wrong?" With the grimace plastered on my face I answered her with another question, "How long have you been like this?" She whispered, "I don't know." She had been walking on shards of a broken beer bottle for days without even knowing it! The only reason she came to the hospital was the fact that an infection had set in and it made her feel sick. As I started to carefully remove each piece of glass with a forceps I asked her if she had ever seen the bottom of her foot. She said no.

Denial can be a terrible companion to disease, especially with diabetes. Some diabetics refuse to recognize that their feet are part of their own bodies. In later stages of the disease, the sensory nerves of the hands and feet are damaged. This is called peripheral neuropathy. The damage can be so severe that the patients have no feeling in their feet at all. Since there is no protective feeling, patients can literally destroy their feet and even walk on broken glass, without feeling a thing. Diabetic neuropathy patients can walk around on crushed bones for weeks and even months. Add to this pathologic process a generous helping of alcoholism and depression and you have the tragic figure that stood before me.

I remembered a pearl from medical school: "Give a man a fish and you feed him for a day. Teach a man to fish and you feed him for a lifetime." The medical corollary is to educate a person to treat their disease. Specifically in diabetics, the patients are taught to respect their extremities because of the lack of protective sensation. They are taught to inspect the bottom of their feet at least once a day. Unfortunately many patients are too old and stiff and can't bend enough to see the bottom of their foot. In these cases patients are instructed to buy a mirror to make the process easier.

Being energetic and committed to fight disease at every street corner, I scampered throughout the hospital looking for a mirror. It was three o'clock in the morning, but I wanted to make a difference and do the right thing. In the back conference room I found a small cosmetic mirror that the nurses would use when they smeared a layer of icing on their faces. I then carefully described diabetic neuropathy to the patient in layman's terms. I thought she was paying very close attention, but she could just have easily been racking her brain as to where she could get a cigarette in the hospital at that time of night. I put the mirror under her foot as the finale to my presentation.

When she saw the mess her foot was in she started to cry hysterically. She let out a howl that would be the envy of the Hound of Baskerville. The horrible mournful noise echoed through the emergency room. Immediately the nurses left their posts behind the potato chip bags and donut boxes and ran into the room. They gave me mean looks and asked me what happened.

The very idea that I could become diabetic was terrifying. I had to beat it. Being a physician I understood a lot about diabetes, but I wanted to know more about the enemy.

If you are not interested in simple facts about early diabetes, you may wish to skip the next two paragraphs. From the Center of Disease Control and Prevention (CDC) web site[5] I gleaned the following:

About Diabetes

- Prediabetes is a term used to identify people who are at increased risk of developing diabetes. People with prediabetes have Impaired Fasting Glucose (IFG) or Impaired Glucose Tolerance (IGT). Some people may have both IFG and IGT.

- IFG is a condition in which the fasting blood sugar level is elevated (100 to 125 milligrams per deciliter or mg/dL) after an overnight fast but is not high enough to be classified as diabetes.

- IGT is a condition in which the blood sugar level is elevated (140 to 199 mg/dL) after a 2-hour oral glucose tolerance test, but is not high enough to be classified as diabetes.

- In a cross-section of U.S. adults aged 40-74 years who were tested from 1988 to 1994, 33.8% had IFG, 15.4% had IGT, and 40.1% had prediabetes (IGT or IFG or both). Were these percentages applied to the 2000 U.S. population, about 35 million adults aged 40-74 would have IFG, 16 million would have IGT, and 41 million would have prediabetes.

- Progression to diabetes among those with prediabetes is not inevitable. Studies suggest that weight loss and increased physical activity among people with prediabetes can prevent or delay diabetes and may return blood glucose levels to normal.

- People with prediabetes are already at increased risk for other adverse health outcomes such as heart disease and stroke.

Research studies have found that lifestyle changes can prevent or delay the onset of Type II Diabetes among high-risk adults. These studies included people with IGT and other high-risk characteristics for developing diabetes. Lifestyle interventions included diet and moderate physical activity (such as walking for 2.5 hours each week). In the Diabetes Prevention Program, a large prevention study of people at high risk for diabetes, such lifestyle interventions reduced the development of diabetes by 58% over 3 years.

I can't remember any other details from my day in the doctor's office, other than the thought in my mind that I had reached rock bottom. At the time, the feeling of rock bottom was concrete and real. I had to do something about it and right away. I had to take it seriously. This had to be it. I didn't realize until months later the metaphysical nature of hitting rock bottom. Each person must have his or her own internal triggers, and being a physician who has taken care of diabetic complications, Type II diabetic onset was mine. Luckily I had recognized rock bottom. Some people never do.

The CDC defines obesity as a body mass index of thirty or greater[6]. During the past 20 years there has been a dramatic increase in obesity in the United States. In 1985 only a few states were participating in the CDC's Behavioral Risk Factor Surveillance System (BRFSS) and providing obesity data. Since then, obesity has become a new national problem of epidemic proportions.

In 1991, four states had obesity prevalence rates of 15–19% and no state had rates at or above 20 percent. In 2004, 7 states had obesity prevalence rates of 15–19%; 33 states had rates of 20–24%; and 9 states had rates more than 25% (no data was available for one state)[7]. The nine states with the highest obesity rates were Michigan, Texas, Louisiana, Alabama, Mississippi, Arkansas, Tennessee, Kentucky and West Virginia.

Clearly weight gain is a problem for many Americans. Knowing the facts is a good start. The next step is what to do about it.

Take-Home Points:

1. **Believe the scale**

2. **Believe the statistics**

3. **Believe the problem exists**

3

The Angry Hungry Man

Once I accepted my weight was a problem, I had to decide how to tackle it. From my medical training I knew that a reasonable sustainable diet was paramount. I was intimidated by the ever growing Obesity Industrial Complex of books, psychologists, physiologists, physicians, intestinal-bypass surgeons, hypnotists, biochemists, nutritionists, self-help groups and dieticians. Where do you start? Should I join a self-help group like Weight-Watchers? Maybe I should sew a big nylon stitch on my lips for a month and drink out of a straw. I even considered having one of the general surgeons cut my bowels and divert the stream of food.

Whenever I face a new problem I try to heed the words of Marcus Aurelius, "Look to the essence of a thing, whether it be a point of doctrine, of practice, or of interpretation[8]."

I realized I was addicted to food, and in great quantities. Everything revolved around the next meal. Where was I going to eat the next meal? What was I going to eat? I bounced between starving and stuffed four or five times a day. Was I going to have enough time to eat today between appointments? If I didn't have time, how could I get something to eat? I need a Coke, give me one of the 20 ouncers. I don't like diet drinks, they taste terrible. Who drinks water? Maybe one of my assistants could run up and buy lunch for the office? Did any of those pharmaceutical salesmen bring any food in today? What's for dessert? Does someone have chocolate? You over there, I know you are a chocolate-hoarder. Open that desk drawer now! Give me some of that salt-water taffy from your beach trip last year, I'll eat anything.

It was crazy. I had to break the addiction, but how?

How would I remove the environmental incentives to eat? I had to fully understand and study the problem before I could fix it.

The Problem With Eating Out

First of all, I had to stop eating out. Everyone knows you overeat when you eat out. Let's take one end of the spectrum: all you can eat, or AUCE, the acronym we used in college. When I say the term AUCE, I think of the last AUCE I had in college. Of course the standard routine was an all-out no-holds-barred eat-off where the winner eats the most food and the loser stops eating or vomits. It's a bad idea no matter what type of food you ingest.

Just examine my favorite restaurant, McDonald's. You're hungry and tired. The kids are in the back seat chanting, "Mickey D's, Mickey D's, Mickey D's." You can't drive more than a mile through any city or suburban sprawl without catching a glimpse of the Golden Arches. The arches speak to me in tongues; they are ever present and enticing. Their allure bypasses the rational cerebral cortex portion of my brain. The arches speak directly to the deepest portions of my brainstem and limbic system that control the basic functions of hunger and memory.

My favorite McDonald's meal[9] is a Double Quarter Pounder with cheese (730 calories), large fries (520 calories) and a large coke (310 calories). Just the thought of it makes me salivate, but more on Pavlov's dogs later. The total calorie count for the meal: 1,560 calories!

And McDonald's is by no means the only place to get a high-calorie meal. How do you limit calories when you eat out for a business dinner? The average portion for most restaurants is probably 1,500 calories per meal. Many restaurants I go to don't even bother listing the nutritional content of the menus on their Web sites. If I was ever served a reasonable portion at a restaurant I would swear to my wife we were ripped off. I would call it all sorts of derogatory names such as "high-falutin," "fru-fru," or "too high class for my tastes," and then leave in a huff, never to return again.

Even worse is going to a relative's house to eat. Growing up in a Greek family, eating reasonably at a meal was just not acceptable behavior. Refusing food immediately brought on an interrogation. I can hear it now in my head: "Don't you want any more food? Did you not like the food? I spent a long time cooking all of the food today, a slave in the kitchen; the least you can do is eat a little more. Did you eat before you came over today? What do you want to eat? If you tell me I will cook it. Don't worry, I'll run out to the grocery store and get you whatever you want. Do you not like my cooking? I know it's not your mother's cooking, but could you please eat some more? Look at your cousin; can't you eat more like him? Are you disgusted with me and my cooking? Are my house and kitchen not clean enough for you? Am I not a clean person? Are you embarrassed to be my guest? Why do you insult our home? Why do you hate me? I will tell your mother about this! Get out! GET OUT!"

Another routine is the parental guilt trip. Eating at my parent's home is always a problem. It starts with a simple reasonable request. "Please finish your plate." Next the level increases. "Okay, we have a little food left in the pot; please finish it off so we don't have to throw it away." The guilt trip comes next. "We paid for this food with hard-earned money, and the least you could do is eat it. Do you know how hard your father has to work to bring home money so we could buy this food for you to eat?" Sometimes we even get the vertical description of the societal food distribution process. "By not finishing this food you disrespect every person involved: the farmer who planted and raised the food, the worker who cultivated, picked it and slaughtered it, the teamster who loaded it on the dock, the captain who piloted the ship through the ocean to bring it, the pilot who flew it to the airport, the truck driver who drove it, the grocer who sold it, and your poor mother who carried it all the way home in a bag to feed you!" And if that didn't sway you there was always the historical comparison. "When I was your age the German army occupied Athens and we were hungry for years! HUNGRY FOR YEARS! When I was five, I had to walk three miles to fill a huge pot with government-provided soup for my entire family! We would steal food by the roadside that fell from the army trucks. You don't know what hunger is!! The children of America are spoiled. You will never know what hunger is!! NEVER!!"

A painful trap I fell into recently was visiting an old friend's house. My former roommate and close friend from surgical residency training had cooked up a storm for dinner. He and his wife were just being hospitable. I tried to resist temptation and timidly ate like a bird. I got nervous when I furtively caught my friend curiously looking at my plate. His one eyebrow was raised and inquisitive. He could sense my fear so I kept my head down and tried to act casual. It didn't work.

First came the taunt: "Is that all you can eat?" Next came the sentimental plea: "Don't you remember how we used to eat on Sunday nights watching football? We made an entire pan of Mousaka for the week and we finished it before EPSN SportsCenter was over." Then came the coup de grace. "Come on, it's just you and me left here now with all of these women and children, and we have two steaks to finish. You and me!"

Within three minutes I smoked down another two-pound Delmonico steak.

Hungry at Home

Avoiding eating away from home is relatively easy: you stop eating out. The behavior that's difficult to break is overeating at home. Let me give you the usual scenario. You had a long day at work and it's time to go home. You're hungry the minute you get in the car. This is the first conditioned stimulus, which triggers the cascade of inappropriate eating. More on behavioral cues later. Just turning the key in the ignition makes you think of food. You make a call, just to see how the kids are doing. At the end of your conversation with your wife, you sheepishly ask if there was anything for dinner tonight. Sadly, this question always comes several blocks prior to the intersection with your favorite pizza place or McDonalds. Once you hear the dinner description, you start to salivate. You get hungrier. The traffic jams and road rage whip your appetite into a fury. You're honking your horn at strangers and flipping the bird to people for cutting you off. By the time you lug your briefcase into your house you're delirious and desperate with hunger.

Halfway down the front hallway you catch a whiff of whatever is cooking. You're so single-minded in your march to the kitchen that you sweep your children aside as they toddle up to greet you. You stumble through the usual obstacle course of discarded toys, crushing some as you go. It only hardens your determination. You open the nearest pot to try and taste whatever's for dinner. You float some type of cliché compliment as a smoke screen. Your wife slaps your hand and says, "Can't you wait for dinner?" You look at her through a squint of anger and rage. Your youngest is pulling on your pant leg and you shake her off, can't deal with anything right now. You run up and change your clothes because you are going to rip through your meal like a linebacker defending the one yard line and you don't want to get the tie stained. By the time your plate hits the table you are eating with such fury your family cringes. Both hands are furiously working at the same time in perfect sync with your ever-grinding jaw. It's poetry in action, the Bolshoi Ballet on steroids. No time to chew or speak. Food gets shoveled in your mouth before you're done chewing the last mouthful. At this point the kids know to keep their distance. You're swallowing things whole: tortellini, meatballs, and olives with the pit still inside. Doesn't matter what it is. Within minutes you're filling your plate with seconds and then thirds. Your wife asks you if you want something to drink and you growl. How can you think of liquid during a famine like this?! You beat the dog to the scrap of food on the floor that the baby dropped over the side of the high chair.

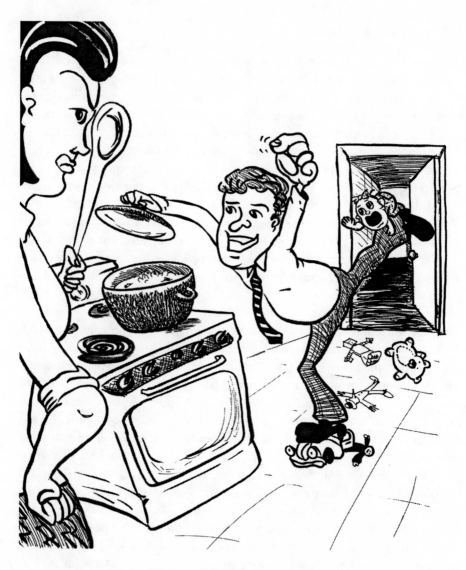

The Angry Hungry Man has arrived.

When the meal is over you excuse yourself to help clean up the dishes and find you're licking dinner remnants from bowls and pots. Once again you have over-eaten. And still, you find yourself scouring the freezer for ice cream or dessert.

It's relatively easy to avoid eating somewhere else, but you can't avoid eating at home. You can, however, control what you eat at home. But first you have to consider what kind of diet you should have and just how much food you should be eating.

The basic measure of energy is the calorie. Food introduces it to your body and exercise and activity liberate it. Any long-term excess energy is stored eventually as adipose fat. A calorie is defined[10] as the amount of heat required to raise the temperature of one kilogram of water one degree centigrade. It also is used as a measure of heat or energy-producing value of food or for a quantity of food having this value. It's relatively easy to assess what your diet should be. The Food and Nutrition Board of the Institute of Medicine National Academies[11] publishes an annual Dietary Reference Intake (DRI's). The DRI explicitly details the exact government suggested diet. In the 2005 table,[12] a 30-year-old 5'11" man with a BMI of 24.99 (is that you?) has a daily caloric requirement of 2,884 calories.

Make no mistake: Diet does matter. In an interesting study, adult rats were placed on a "supermarket diet"[13] consisting of chocolate chip cookies, salami, cheese, bananas, marshmallows, milk chocolate, peanut butter, sweetened condensed milk and fat. Is this diet familiar to you? A control rat group also had access to all you can eat laboratory chow (sounds boring). The supermarket rats gained a whopping 269% more weight than the controls in two months time.

How do you control your eating and diet to lose weight? I always want to strangle those smug friends who repeat the obvious simplistic mantra: It's all about calories in and calories out. There's more to it of course. How do you motivate yourself to follow the mantra and put it into effect? What's the catalyst to change? That's where the hot sauce diet comes into play.

Take-Home Points:

1.   **Understand your behaviors**

2.   **Avoid behavioral cues**

3.   **Your behaviors must change**

4

How is Hot Sauce Going to Help?

One of my most enjoyable medical school classes at Johns Hopkins was psychiatry. The chairman at the time, Dr. Paul McHugh, required our class to read his textbook, <u>The Perspectives of Psychiatry</u>[14]. My initial impression was of someone tooting his own horn by making us read his book. I went on to read the book three times that year for the shear pleasure of it. The premise of the book was that the field of psychiatry has four perspectives: Disease, Dimensions, Life Experience and Behavior. The Disease perspective is one of medical diagnosis, chemical and anatomical details, medicines, etc. The Dimensions perspective identifies a continuum of personality traits for each individual. The Life Experience perspective involves overlaying the literal life story of an individual with what happened in life and how they responded or adapted. The final perspective—Behavior—suggests that people's actions are based on behaviors, basically stimulus and response.

The scope of this chapter is not, by any means, to cover and understand psychiatry, but rather to illustrate my story of coping with my personal problem of obesity by using my limited knowledge of medicine with the hope it helps someone else. First, I need to cover some behavioral basics.

Behavioral Conditioning

There are some things about behavior I understand. Let's take my upbringing for example. My mother's upbringing was agrarian and rough. Stubborn mules were whipped. Dogs were kept outside and fed only scraps. Children were seen and not heard. Bad children were punished by spanking. I always knew that unruly behavior would meet with a slap of my mother's hand. I can picture the hand now, strong from an upbringing of farm chores. On the back of it was her wedding ring of gold and a massive cubic zirconia she would show off to the rich old ladies in our church. Getting spanked really hurt, especially if I got clocked in the face with the ring. Punishment definitely worked. This is what eventually inspired me to use hot sauce to control my behaviors. I understand this perspective of psychiatry is pedestrian to most. Needless to say my children only get the chair time-out. I use hot sauce as a punishment, as adverse conditioning. Although hot sauce is pungent, I do also enjoy it. I'm not alone, hot sauce is popular.

I'd like to give a little background on conditioning. In his study of physiology, Ivan Pavlov (1849-1936) performed surgery on dogs[15] so that their salivary glands excreted fluid out of the cheeks instead of into the mouth. He could easily observe their glands this way. He then gave stimuli to them that caused salivation: the sight of food, the sound of food coming by the experimenter, etc. These stimuli caused salivation, as you would expect. These normal stimuli and responses are unconditioned stimuli and responses. Pavlov then associated these normal stimuli of food with a metronome that the dogs would hear. The metronome was a conditioned stimulus. After some time, if the dogs would hear the metronome by itself, they would be fooled into thinking food was coming and would salivate. This is a conditioned response to a conditioned stimulus. Eventually if you stopped associating the metronome with food, they would learn and stop salivating to the metronome. This is called extinction. Another example of extinction is a baby crying at night. The baby expects the mother to answer the cry and pick him or her up. The stimulus is crying and the response is the mother picking up the baby. When the mother stops picking the baby up at night, the crying to be picked up eventually stops. This is extinction of the behavior. The first few nights are very rough and most parents have to deal with more than the usual share of crying. This is called an extinction burst. Every parent can relate.

This reminds me of a story of my fraternity house years and our cook, Blanche. She hated it when we were in our kitchen. She chased us out with anything she could find. Her weapons were shouts followed by a knife, frying pan, or skillet. Initially she would scream for us to come down, "Dinner's ready!" A stampede of twenty-five fools would run her over every day. The food sometimes would run out, as there were serious appetites in the house. We ran and roughhoused to the food line to make sure we got our fair share. Once she was almost knocked to the ground. She learned her lesson. From that day forth she developed a new technique. She would get dinner completely ready and get dressed to go home. On the way out she would ring the house fire alarm and run like the devil. We soon realized that three rings was the signal for dinner and we would drop everything and run. As you might imagine, it wasn't long before the bell would make us salivate.

To test behaviors B.F. Skinner (1904-1990)[16] created an operant chamber later called the Skinner Box. A hungry (80% body weight) or thirsty animal (i.e. pigeon) is placed in a box and is required to press a bar to obtain food or water. Behaviors could be "shaped" in steps. An example of the rewarded steps is: #1 reward looking at illuminated yellow key; #2 reward approaching illuminated yellow key; #3 reward putting beak on yellow key; and #4 reward for a peck on the key. BF Skinner wrote,

> "Operant conditioning behaviors are a function of an organism's history of reinforcement; a self or personality is at best a repertoire of behavior imparted by an organized set of contingencies."

Punishment is an aversive stimulus that should decrease a response. Unfortunately, sometimes punishment can provoke counter-aggression. Punishment for a certain behavior can also be described as aversive conditioning.

Below is a table summarizing Skinner's findings:

NATURE OF STIMULUS

	Positive	Negative
Presentation of behavior involved	Positive Reinforcement (increases the behavior)	Punishment (decreases the behavior)
Removal of behavior involved	Punishment (decreases the behavior)	Negative Reinforcement (increases the behavior)

I could clearly understand how behavior works. I knew my behavior was one of inappropriate hunger, disproportionate portion sizes and excessive caloric consumption. Does this sound familiar to you? I was eating like a starved maniac. I was conditioned to become hungry from driving home in my car, opening the door to my house, preparing food, and looking at the food in the pot. The way I ate was fast and furious. In my haste I didn't taste my food. I usually swallowed it whole like a snake.

First, I wanted to punish my inappropriate hunger. It wasn't right for me to feel the way I did. I decided to use hot sauce. Like many, I've always liked it. Whenever I feel the uncontrollable urge to eat voraciously I give myself a slap of hot sauce. We'll get into the details later. When I'm uncontrollably starving, I generously cover my food with it. Every meal is nice and spicy. The hot sauce slap tames my hunger, slows down my eating, and encourages me to drink several glasses of water with my meal. Within minutes, the irresistible urge to eat is gone.

Second, I needed to change the way I ate.

The Active Ingredient: Capsaicin

Let's get back to hot sauce for a moment so we can fully understand it. Many are afraid of hot sauce and cringe at the thought of applying it liberally. Let me be the first to say that the only thing we have to fear in hot sauce is fear itself.

The active ingredient of hot sauce is capsaicin[17]. Capsaicin is derived from the capsicum plant and is specifically a mixture of intensely pungent compounds called capsaicinoids. Capsaicin is extremely potent. Capsicum pepper imparts a pungent taste to water even when diluted one part in 11 million parts water[18]. Capsaicin causes an initial aversive response of a burn-like sensation in the mouth and throat, flushing of the face and neck and sweating of the forehead. The preference for hot sauce cannot be established in an animal model and is an exclusively adult acquired taste. One description[17] of the allure of hot sauce is

> "A thrill seeking masochism meeting the challenge of explosive sensory response overcoming the initial negative effects to enjoy the high sense of relief."

Why not punish yourself in other ways, like the self-flagellating John Savage of Huxley's <u>Brave New World</u>? How about biting your lip, setting your hand over a candle flame or threading needles through your skin? There are many reasons to use hot sauce.

The use of hot sauce is socially accepted, easily titrated, safe, effective, and an inducement to drink water. Like cigarette smoking or illicit drugs, food can be an addictive substance. However, unlike them it cannot be completely avoided or removed. Food must be controlled and managed. What better way to control it than a socially accepted spice that stimulates the same nerve pathways as food? Titration is simple; you just keep adding more until it works for you.

Hot sauce is an accepted food additive or spice and it's cheap. Capsaicin's earliest use[17] was as a food additive in Mexico and South America. It can make a monotonous diet interesting. A bottle of hot spice costs less than $5 dollars and can be found in almost any cafeteria, restaurant or grocery store. Hot sauce is accepted by society, so there is no stigma associated with its use. I would never in a million years drink a can of the latest "diet plan milkshake". Dosing myself with a helping of hot sauce makes me feel like a tough guy, not an effeminate woman with a diet shake drink. When I'm at the dinner table with my family or friends I use hot sauce with pride. When my face flushes red it's my red badge of courage.

In fact, people who see me piling on the hot sauce frequently come up to me during lunch and whisper in my ear that they are big hot sauce fans as well. You'll be part of the hot sauce secret society. The occasional hot sauce consumer who uses it in moderation may even have great respect for you. I occasionally get compliments from people who are so impressed they shout out, "Wow, you can really put on the hot sauce!" or "How can you eat so much hot sauce?" There is absolutely nothing embarrassing associated with using hot sauce. No one will realize you are using it to diet, so there is no dieting stigma. You won't have to explain why you are dieting. This way you avoid all of the ridiculous annoying comments such as "You don't need to lose weight" or "How much do you weigh and how much do you want to lose?" Worst of all is the diet authority who scoffs at your dieting attempts. The diet authority always enters a long painful editorial monologue on how to lose weight and how the whole thing works, i.e. calories in and out, blah, blah, blah. If someone suspects you are trying to lose weight you can laugh at them sardonically through a mirror-rehearsed sneer and say "Nonsense, I like the taste!" Your weight loss program is performed in secret right under everyone's noses.

How To Use Hot Sauce

Let's get down to the nitty-gritty. How do you do it? How do you use it? Hot sauce can be titrated to meet your needs. Use just enough for it to work for you. Everyone has variations in taste bud sensitivity and therefore the dosage should be increased for those with less sensitive taste buds and decreased for those with sensitive ones. I categorize the dosages in three ways: mild "flavoring," moderate "pushback," and aggressive "blowout."

"Flavoring" is the mildest form of hot sauce use and the most commonly used. As an example, for lunch I have a small bowl of soup and a turkey burger. We'll get into the details of how to eat in the next chapter. I mete out the hot sauce dosage such that the soup takes me exactly ten minutes to eat. I wear a watch at all times to keep an eye on the time while I eat. My favorite soup is tomato as I feel it mixes well with hot sauce. If you are eating it faster put some more hot sauce in, if slower ease up on it the next day. The amount of hot sauce should also encourage you to drink a good amount of water. Don't be afraid to drink water, it's good for you and it's one of the few things that has no calories. You need to drink water while you eat. You may say, "I just can't get myself to drink the water

I'm supposed to drink." It is difficult, but once the hot sauce starts burning your mouth, the water will provide you an oasis of comfort. Slowly drink the soup or eat your food and feel the hot sauce working on your taste buds. If you don't drink the water while you eat, the hot sauce diet simply won't work. You have to feel the burn and drink the water to make the diet work.

How much water should you drink? The 2005 Dietary Reference Intake[11] recommends 3.7 liters of water or fluid a day for a 35-year-old-male. I'm convinced many people eat food when they are thirsty. I know I do. To get a reference, one cup equals 8 ounces, which equals 236 milliliters or a quarter liter. Doing the math, that means you need 15 cups of water per day. Personally, I drink two cups of coffee in the morning. Being a surgeon, I shared the old-school football coach mentality of rarely giving myself water breaks. I couldn't take breaks during surgery and I never took water breaks in the office until all the work was done. Don't be a foolish coach, frequently take water breaks. That brings us to lunch.

I buy two 20-ounce diet sodas, diet drinks or waters. It can be tough balancing the drinks on your cafeteria tray, but after a while you'll be a pro at it. Fluids laced with high caloric fructose are unnecessary and not an option. Make sure you look at the label to make sure there are no calories in the drink. That should be 1 liter for lunch. This might raise some suspicion amongst your lunch partners but can be easily brushed off with the curt response "I'm thirsty". The soup should be titrated with hot sauce so that the first 20 ounces of water is comfortably consumed to quench the heat from the soup. Again this should take ten minutes. The second 20 ounces can be consumed with the rest of lunch or later that afternoon. Spicing the turkey burger is optional depending on your hunger and self-control. If you are able to drink the two waters and consume your reasonably portioned lunch in a minimum of 20 minutes you are a lunch graduate of the hot sauce diet. Once you have graduated you will always be an alumnus, and you will certainly need to go back to school occasionally for relapses of poor eating behavior. You know what to do, it's easy. The goal is to sustain a lifetime of normal eating behaviors and not to suck down gallons of hot sauce.

Dinner should be flavored in a very similar way to lunch to slow down your meal to a minimum of 20 minutes and to ensure that you drink at least two 20-ounce fluid servings. One can easily adjust the amount of hot sauce in your food so that you will drink one to three glasses of water, and just enough to slow you down while eating. If you can adhere to this schedule you have met 80% of your daily fluid requirements. Mild hot sauce flavoring may be all you need to adhere to your diet. If not, more aggressive measures can be taken.

Pushbacks and Blowouts

Recall the hungry man coming home from work scenario described in Chapter 3. Scary isn't it? The hungry man coming home from work is stronger and faster than an experienced NFL linebacker hunting down his prey. He can rip through 1,000 calories of cheese, chips, and the family's dinner before he even lets go of his briefcase. The hungry man needs to be pushed back by something as strong and immobile as an offensive tackle. The inappropriate hunger behavior needs to be punished with a "pushback."

The mild usual "pushback" form is a cup of tomato juice with hot sauce titrated so that the need for immediate food is removed. The titration should also encourage drinking water to start on the minimum of two 20 ounces of fluid for dinner. If you find your hand wandering towards the cookie jar or cheese drawer in the fridge you need to get a more serious dose of the pushback. For serious inappropriate uncontrollable hunger, I recommend a full swig of hot sauce straight from the bottle. I know this is drastic, but inappropriate hunger behavior needs to be punished. Once the swig is in your mouth, you should not swallow it immediately but rather swish it around like a wine connoisseur until the burning effect diminishes. I didn't say it would be easy. My reasoning will be given in the next several paragraphs. Think of it as a slow swish and swallow. That's right; it has to be done for the good of your health and society. You should feel the immediate pungency of the capsaicin and reach for the water bottle and hopefully down a large glass of water. If this fails try another swig. If this fails you need the atom bomb or "blowout."

The "blowout" should be used sparingly as I feel it has the highest potential for counter-aggression and non-compliance with the hot sauce diet. For the blowout you may need to have several hot chili peppers on standby from the grocery store. The blowout should be enough hot sauce in the form of a large swig or hot peppers to make you grab a massive glass of water and evacuate the kitchen immediately. The blowout should force you to drink several consecutive glasses of ice water to quench the burning as you head for the hills. You should feel the burning in your mouth and face as if you received a slap for misbehavior. Remember that it's punishment for inappropriate behavior, you really deserve this. Another alternative to quench the burning is an ice cube in the mouth between glasses of water. The blowout should knock out your appetite for good. In the first month of the hot sauce diet I personally required two blowouts a week to stop my inappropriate food-seeking behavior. I've also used the blowout to immediately stop several passionate occurrences of the "late-night-eats." The memory keeps me out of the kitchen late at night. The blowout should be used very cautiously and sparingly. There are some potential risks associated with hot peppers and capsaicin.

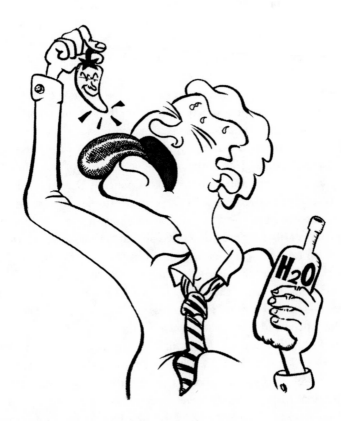

When all else fails to deter overeating, use the blowout.

Is it Safe?

Hot sauce is reasonably safe but massive doses can be dangerous. The effects are seen only when the spice contacts and stimulates taste buds in the mouth[17]. Encapsulated doses of capsaicin do not cause pungent reactions. If the mouth is bypassed in the act of eating hot sauce, the pungent effect doesn't happen. This is the reasoning behind the swish and swallow technique of the pushback. If one performs the swish and swallow correctly, this maximizes the pungency effect and therefore minimizes the hot sauce dose. Minimizing the dose minimizes any health risk associated with hot sauce capsaicin.

In a human subject[17] study 10 grams of ground fresh chilies were mixed with 100 milliliters of water and inserted into the stomach of study participants with the use of a tube from the nose to the stomach (nasogastric tube). The tube bypassed the mouth so that the participants could tolerate a massive dose of hot peppers. The stomach lining of each study subject was then carefully examined with the use of a fiber optic camera (Esophagoduodenoscopy, or EGD). The stomach lining did have evidence of edema and in some cases bleeding. Bypassing the mouth removes the protective pungent effect of capsaicin.

In an unusual toxicology study[18] performed at the Duquesne University School of Pharmacy in Pittsburgh, researchers studied the effects of massive doses of Tabasco® sauce given to lab rats. The premise of the study was to find the LD_{50} dose of a common commercial hot sauce. LD_{50}: (Lethal Dose 50)[19] is the dose of a chemical which kills 50% of a sample population. Such values are widely reported and used as an effective measure of the potential toxicity of chemicals. Various massive doses of Tabasco® sauce were inserted into the stomachs of lab rats with the use of a tube to bypass the mouth (orogastric intubation). As a fellow student of science I apologize to all of the animal rights sympathizers who are cringing at the thought. This model is obviously not how we ingest hot sauce. The rats were then given access to food and water and observed. All rats were sacrificed and their anatomy was studied.

Out of thirty seven rat deaths all but three occurred within 24 hours and the balance in 72 hours. The rats who died showed signs of hypothermia (low body temperature), tachypnea (accelerated breathing rate), and lethargy. The gastrointestinal tracts of the rats were studied post-mortem and interestingly there were no ulcerations, perforations, or bleeding in the esophagus, stomach and intestines. The LD_{50} in male rats was 23 ml/kg. The dose for females was similar. Other than occasional diarrhea there were no anatomical abnormalities noted in the brain, heart, lung, liver, kidney, spleen, stomach, and intestine of any of the rats. If you extrapolated to a 154 lb human adult this would be a whopping 1.4 liters or a third of a gallon of Tabasco® sauce all at once. The mere thought of such a thing gives me indigestion. Fortunately, the pungency of the capsaicin in hot sauce will prevent excessive doses. When people eat hot sauce, it's never with a tube to bypass the mouth. It would defeat the purpose of hot sauce.

The last few paragraphs were a bit scary, but must be kept in perspective. The way the hot sauce was inserted into the people and rats was unnatural. Ingesting massive amounts of hot sauce does not happen in real life. The main question many people ask is, "Won't I get heartburn or an ulcer by eating so much hot sauce?" This is a very good question. When I first got started I thought I would get heartburn or an ulcer. The diet was working so I bit the bullet and rolled the dice. In my mind it was going to be a calculated risk I had to take. Desperate times necessitated desperate measures. To my surprise absolutely nothing bad happened. I read up on peptic ulcer disease and spicy food and the evidence was unequivocally clear: there was no link between spicy food and ulcers.

In a recent gastrointestinal textbook[20] the author states:

> "No study has established a convincing link between diet and peptic ulcer disease (PUD). Patients often describe indigestion associated with the ingestions of certain foods (e.g. spicy foods), but the evidence that such foods cause ulceration is virtually nonexistent. Bland diets have not been shown to have any benefit in preventing or treating PUD."

> "Despite the observation[21] that some types of foods and beverages are reported to cause indigestion, there are no convincing data indicating that any specific diet causes ulcers. The factors responsible for indigestions associated with highly spiced foods are unknown. Although bland meals and the frequent ingestion of milk were commonplace in the armamentarium of ulcer treatment in the early 1900's, they neither expedite ulcer healing nor prevent recurrences or complications. Dietary alterations, other than instructions to avoid pain-causing foods, are unnecessary for ulcer patients."

I will not engage the exact details of what type of diet to use. If you are unsure what a balanced diet is, I suggest a start by reading our government's recommendations[22]. *Dietary Guidelines for Americans* is published jointly every 5 years by the Department of Health and Human Services (HHS) and the Department of Agriculture (USDA). The *Guidelines* provide authoritative advice for people about how good dietary habits can promote health and reduce the risk of major chronic diseases. If this is too long or boring there are a zillion books on the subject in any neighborhood bookstore or website. Several free National Institute of Health (NIH) web sites are very helpful and user friendly, try http://www.nhlbisupport.com/chd1/lifestyles.htm and http://www.nhlbi.nih.gov.

Facts About Food

Three important facts about food content need to be remembered while dieting; you can't win with hot sauce alone. You also need to use some common sense.

The three most common components of food[23] are carbohydrates (4.2kcal/gram), protein (5.65 kcal/gram), and lipids (9.45 kcal/gram). The benefits of limiting high caloric fat and the metabolic need for protein are obvious. Everyone knows weight loss and getting in shape are best accomplished with diet and exercise. What about cutting out the carbs? The problem with removing carbohydrates from your diet is that they are essential in improving your physical performance. Glycogen is the energy source for muscles in aerobic activity.

Carbohydrates are saccharides[24]. Simple forms are monosaccharides and disaccharides such as sucrose, lactose and maltose. Sucrose is the component of cane sugar and is comprised of glucose and fructose. Complex carbohydrates are polysaccharides and are starches such as wheat, peas, corn and beans, as well as pasta (my favorite) and rice. The circulating energy source of your body is Glucose-6-Phosphate. The majority of carbohydrates in a healthy diet should be complex types such as pasta, bread, and high caloric vegetables. Glucose-6-Phosphate is converted and stored in your body as glycogen. If there are excess carbohydrates in your bloodstream beyond the immediate energy needs of your body and storage depots the body stores them as triglycerides in adipose or fat. Go ahead and feel your belly. Do you have enough energy stores to heat Madison Square Garden?

When your body exercises it needs energy. The first level of energy source while exercising is the glucose in your blood. Blood glucose can supply 4 to 5 grams of glucose or 20 calories. The next two sources of energy are from glycogen stores and these are stored in your liver and muscle. Your liver contains approximately 75 to100 grams of glycogen or 300 to 400 calories. Your muscle mass contains 13 to 15 grams/kg of muscle, so depending on your muscle mass you have 375 to 450 grams of glycogen in your muscles or 1,500 to 1,800 calories.

Fatigue during exercise is in large part due to carbohydrate deficiency. As is detailed above, muscle glycogen stores are the major energy source in prolonged periods of maximal aerobic exercise. Let's assume walking burns approximately 100 calories per mile for an average 154 lb (70 kg) thin person and that there are 8 city blocks per mile. Your blood glucose is gone by the first 2 blocks. Your liver energy stores are spent after 3 to 4 miles. After that point you're relying on the store of glycogen in your muscles. Muscle glycogen stores therefore limit serious exercise. The greater the level of aerobic fitness, the greater the ability to synthesize muscle glycogen. It's an important component to reaching peak aerobic physical fitness.

Having understood the need for glycogen to get in good aerobic physical shape, how can you cut carbs completely out of your diet? You should not. Of course this is not a free get-out-of-carb-jail card into a spaghetti orgy. Carbs still contain calories and they can very easily put you over your caloric limit. One must always remember the teachings of ancient Greece, "Moderation in all things."

Low-carb diet fads frequently disregard basic nutritional principles of balance, variety and moderation[2]. Low-carb diets can cause a person to urinate water, so half of the initial weight loss can be explained by a loss of total body water.

Researchers[25] compared a low-carb, mixed, and high-carb diet in a group of human subjects. A high-carb diet was directly proportional with increased glycogen content in the quadriceps muscle of the thigh. A high-carb diet approximately tripled the duration of exercise endurance as measured on a bicycle ergometer (from 60 to 180 minutes). Carbs help you exercise for a long time to get in shape and to lose weight.

Dieting Success

Four diet factors have been associated with long-term success[26,27]: self-monitoring, stimulus control, reinforcement of eating and exercise behaviors, and techniques in the act of eating. The last three will be discussed in the next chapter. Each person needs to monitor his or her diet. I don't think this means that every last calorie needs to be counted and logged. I do think that everyone should know exactly what they do eat. The FDA (Food and Drug Administration)[28] requires that all food manufacturers list their products' ingredients and nutritional information on the food label. It's so easy to turn around every jar, can or package and read the calorie content. Once you start doing it, you'll never stop. It's interesting and you'll learn a lot. This is not an obsessive eating behavior but rather an educational practice to know what you eat. Don't be fooled by the sample servings. I generally multiply the calorie per serving by the servings to find out how many calories are in the entire product. It's important to know how much is in the entire package because usually you eat the whole thing. You should have an idea of how many calories you eat at every meal and every snack. You will be surprised by your efforts. Ballpark your daily calorie consumption to be less than what is suggested by the suggested daily requirement for your age, height and weight.

The act of counting calories is unpleasant. I was at a friend's house for lunch one weekend and I couldn't believe the quality and quantity of the feast the hosts had prepared. I filled my plate to the brim and immediately the host came over and made the motion of a counting machine to count up the calories. I understood at that moment the problem of counting calories. It takes the magical fun out of eating. Eating becomes an accounting exercise with rules and regulations. The act of responsible counting takes away from the pleasure of carefree consumption. In my mind it's an even deeper reminder of our fallibility, physical and mental weaknesses and ultimate mortality as humans. It's a reminder of the human condition. I'll never forget my son's first asthma attack and listening to his hurried breath sounds and rapid heartbeat for the first time. It saddened me to acknowledge that he was a patient, just another physiological machine. His existence had always been categorized in my mind as some sort of supernatural gift. Unfortunately, the reality is that one must be responsible for our actions here on earth, so the calories must be counted to maintain a reasonable body weight. Anything short of counting calories for most people is irresponsible behavior.

Do weigh yourself. Beware: the scale is only a mechanical device and it does not lie. Some scales are more specific than others, but they all operate in a range of accuracy. Believe the number on the scale. If the number on the scale does not decrease or actually increases, the scale is probably not broken or inaccurate. It's your weight at that point in time. If the scale measurement is higher than you want—you are in luck, it can and will go down in time. I personally weigh myself at the same time everyday.

Take Home Points:

1. **Count your calories and know the details of your diet**

2. **Slap the Angry Hungry Man with some hot sauce**

3. **Let the hot sauce work, drink a lot of water to remove the burn**

4. **Eat a balanced, sensible diet**

5

A New Game Plan

As discussed previously, the problem with overeating is that the addictive substance (food) cannot be cut out of your life like cigarettes, alcohol, or illicit drugs. Major therapeutic issues in addiction[27] involve: denial, concomitant psychiatric ailments, matching the treatment to the individual, controlling the behavior, motivation, and relapse.

When I reached rock bottom I finally realized the depths of my denial. As you remember from Chapter 2 I had an excuse and a reason for everything. The large prominent belly was useful as a mobile writing desk. Everyone my age has a belly; it's the middle-aged American way. The scale must be inaccurate. The scale reading is off because I'm wearing heavy clothes. The scale is meaningless because I usually don't weigh this much. I choose to be overweight. This is my personal preference.

Controlling your surrounding stimuli[27] is important in controlling your behaviors. If you are trying to quit smoking, would you take your afternoon break in the outdoor smoking area of your building? Simple restrictions can make a difference.

Be aware of your surroundings and actions just before you eat something. Eat in the same room and the same time every day for each meal. Don't eat over the kitchen sink or in a hallway. Sit down at the dining room or cafeteria table. Don't eat out of the pot or serving bowl. How will you have any idea of how much you are eating unless it's in front of you on a plate? Don't multitask while you're eating. Reading the paper or a book or watching television may be interesting but it also may persuade you to inhale your lunch, and then some. Clear the food off the table after you eat to avoid unnecessary second helpings. When you clean up the kitchen at night avoid scavenging through your daughter's unfinished plate. Just throw the food away. The cost of overeating is always greater than the monetary loss of the food. Don't keep junk food readily available in your house or work place—it will tempt you. Throw the junk food or left-over dessert in the trash. Refuse unnecessary lunches or dinners where you will probably be enticed by massive restaurant portions. While in a restaurant request a meal that fits within the confines of your diet. When someone encourages you to eat more, change the subject. Avoid eating with people who overeat or who eat too fast. You may mimic their actions and go over to the dark side.

Once you start eating, you need to control the act of eating. Try to make every meal last longer than 20 minutes. Hog the conversation if you have to. Avoid multitasking while you eat. Eat with one hand at a time. Swallow each mouthful before you insert the next one. Chew and taste your food. Take a two minute break while eating. Get up from the table if you have to. I call it the two minute drill. During the two minute drill finish a glass of water and get another glass. Avoid the second helping if you can.

Take Home Points:

1. **No more excuses, you are in denial**

2. **Change the way you eat**

3. **Control your environment**

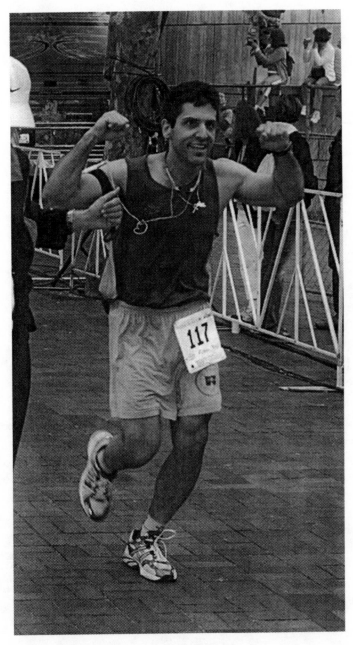

Crossing the May 2006 Flying Pig finish "Swine Line."

6

Training

The ancient Greeks believed in the motto "Sound mind in a sound body." Effective behavioral therapies in weight loss programs[29] share certain attributes: spouse support, strong contingencies, appetite suppressants, length of treatment (minimum 10-12 weeks), and exercise. The first two attributes will be covered in Chapter 7, Motivation. The only appetite suppressant that can be recommended safely is a reasonable dose of coffee. Exercise is a key element to success.

The 2005 Dietary Guidelines[30] recommend 60 minutes of moderate to vigorous activity per day to help manage body weight. According to 2000 data[31], approximately 10% of Americans walk 30 minutes a day for 5 days a week. In 2004 an estimated 423,000 (0.14% of the population) people completed a marathon in the US[32]. An exercise regimen also ensures the weight you lose is fat and not muscle.

I had every excuse in the book for not exercising. My favorite sports have always been basketball and weightlifting. They obviously had failed me. It was difficult getting to the gym. Once at the gym I had to wait to get into a game. Once in the game, sometimes I lost and had to wait until our team was next. I frequently was injured. Sometimes the hand injuries gave me difficulties in my work as a surgeon. I had to compensate with my other hand until I recovered. I went to the gym one or two times a week at best. I was too busy. I had to work early in the morning and I couldn't get to the gym on time to exercise. I had to be fresh at work for surgeries. I started my cases at 7:30 a.m. so I believed there was no way I could exercise in the morning. Once I was home my kids would pummel me with hugs and kisses. I didn't have the heart to leave the house once they saw me.

Get A Move On

Everyone must exercise. The human body was designed and evolved to walk daily. The American Academy of Orthopaedic Surgeons uses the motto "Life is Motion, Motion is Life." Fossils reveal skeletal remains of humans very similar to modern man that are at least 100,000 years old. Human physiology is made to run. Man has been a sedentary creature only in the last 100 years of existence. Our current lifestyle has been in effect only in the last 1/1000 of our existence on the earth as a species at a conservative estimate. It's unnatural not to run, walk, or exercise. Unfortunately our short term existence and immediate needs don't depend on physical activity.

A good exercise program is one you can do at home[33]. Walking is by far the easiest activity in regards to very low injury rate, good physical benefit, and convenience. A 200-pound man burns approximately 133 calories per mile[34]. One hour of walking at a moderate pace of 3 miles an hour will burn approximately 400 calories. Of course, the calories expended in exercise pale in comparison to the calories one can consume within ten minutes. For example a reasonably small piece of cheese cake can be consumed within thirty seconds. It would take an entire hour of walking to expend the same calories. Don't be discouraged. The margins of weight loss are small but ever present in someone who can be disciplined. A small 10% reduction in daily calories (280 calories) over two weeks is a pound of weight loss (one pound equals 3,500 calories).

Walking is an extremely social activity if you find a good friend or partner. Finding a walking partner is relatively easy as most people walk at the same pace, unlike running. Walking injuries are rare. The most common complaints are usually degenerative complaints of the lower back and legs associated more with degenerative arthritis conditions than injuries from the sport.

I try to learn something from every patient I interview and examine. Most often the lesson is useful. One patient was an elderly man with a chief complaint of "mild low back pain." He appeared very neat and fit. Although he was thin, he did have good muscle tone and walked with a normal brisk gait. His mood was cheerful. When I glanced at his age in the chart I was shocked to see he was 93! He looked to be in his sixties. His favorite sports had been football and baseball as a young man. I was intrigued by his story. He stated as he became older he switched to jogging and then walking. He currently walked 30 to 60 minutes a day. I asked him what was the secret to longevity and he said, "Exercise in the morning before your wife and kids wake up."

Exercising in the morning has many benefits. In the warmer months, you avoid the heat and humidity. There is no one to distract you or detain you as everyone is asleep. It is extraordinarily rare to have an emergency to attend to in the morning. In the afternoon and evening they are common and unavoidable. You don't have to fight the food trap in the morning, the devil on the shoulder that hisses, "Just eat dinner and blow off running." There is nothing on your mind to distract you. During the rest of the day, you don't have the sword of Damocles hanging over your head; you have already completed your task. The entire day has a lower level of stress and anxiety as you already completed your daily stress reliever. Your spouse and children aren't wondering where you are and why you're not with them. You don't cancel running for dinner at a nice restaurant for a late meeting (which is an interception run back for a touchdown for the bad guys). The only challenge is going to bed early enough to stay fresh.

Getting Started

In the beginning I started with walking 2 miles a day in the morning. Yes, I was embarrassed that I couldn't run. It was a lumbering jog with breaks of walking on the hills. I tried running but it was too difficult. I wasn't losing weight and I wasn't getting faster. This went on for many months. I was frustrated. Then I hit rock bottom in the doctor's office and I decided to resort to the hot sauce diet in desperation. The diet worked and I lost ten pounds after several weeks. I ran one day with my practice partner and running mentor Dr. Charles Edwards II. Charles has run eight marathons to date and runs with me for encouragement. Charles runs like the latest model of machine in Terminator 2. After losing the first ten pounds, I ran the two miles faster and easier than I ever had before. Weight loss was the key ingredient to running well. I pronounced my new discovery to Charles that weight loss improves running and he looked at me as if I had told him one plus one equaled two. Seeing an opening, Charles then challenged me to run the Annapolis Ten Mile Race, which was four months away at the time. I had never run more than 5 to 6 miles in my life. Running had always been a punishment in the sports I played. I committed to it not knowing if I could do it. Since then I've been running five days a week, averaging 25 miles a week.

With its efficiency, convenience, and low rate of injury, running is very similar to walking. It can also be performed close to home. It can be social or solitary. One mile of running for a 200-pound man burns 136 calories[35] with little relative variance with respect to speed. The caloric expenditures of running and walking over a distance are similar but the biggest difference is time. Six miles can easily be covered in an hour of moderate running, as compared to three miles at a reasonable walking pace. The caloric expenditure is double in the same time period. In one hour I could burn 800 calories. Now we're talking! For anyone interested in reading about the benefits of running, read Jim Fixx's classic book[35] <u>The Complete Book of Running</u>.

Bicycling is an excellent non-weight bearing sport with excellent cardiovascular benefits. Bicycling a moderate 14-miles-per-hour burns approximately 700 calories an hour. Although the energy expenditure is similar to running there are several restrictions and concerns. Bicycling can be weather dependent. Bicycling on a road with cars can be dangerous. In a study from the Wisconsin Bureau of Health Information[36], cycling accounted for a hospitalization rate for injuries of 6.2/100,000 people. The only sports/recreational-related injury that occurred more often was being struck by or against an object in a sport (6.4/100,000).

Bicycling was one of my favorite activities during medical school and orthopaedic residency. After treating several severely injured patients who had been struck by cars while road cycling, my enthusiasm waned. Although the exercise itself is safe in a vacuum, falls and accidents involving automobiles can be disabling and deadly. In my single life these relative risks were acceptable. As a father they are difficult to defend in my mind. An estimated 69,000 traumatic head injuries related to cycling were treated by emergency rooms[37] in the US in 2004. Cycling was the most common mechanism of head injury followed by All Terrain Vehicles (27,000), football (25,000) and basketball (24,000). Although sports injuries contribute to fatalities infrequently, the leading cause of death from sports-related injuries is traumatic brain injury.

Excuses, Excuses

What about the exercise excuses? Listed below, Benjamin Franklin's Poor Richard's Almanac has a good answer for every one of them.

Excuse #1: I don't have time in the morning.

Answer: "No gains without pains." I pushed back my surgical and office hours start time to 8:00 a.m., making morning exercise convenient. I work a little less and I have accepted a small decrease in income. You can't afford *not* to exercise. There should be absolutely no excuse why every person cannot exercise sixty minutes every morning.

Excuse #2: I'm too sleepy in the morning.

Answer: "He that riseth late must trot all day, and shall scarce overtake his business at night." House curfew is a strict 9:00 p.m. for the entire household. The wake-up bugle trumpets at 5:00 a.m. for me and running commences at 5:45 a.m. sharp.

Excuse #3: I have to have my coffee and morning bowel movement prior to exercise (this is my brother's favorite).

Answer: "Who is strong? He that can conquer his bad Habits." Keep a strict time schedule for exercise, bedtime and wake-up time. Your bodily functions will quickly adapt to the new strict train schedule.

Excuse #4: Running is boring.

Answer: "Up, sluggard and waste not life; in the grave will be sleeping enough." Run with headphones and music. Keep the music current. Buy an iPod or the equivalent. The music can motivate you and you won't hear your labored breathing on the hills. Run with different friends and groups. Vary your route. Exercise each day with a different friend. Keep your exercise time consistent.

Excuse #5: I lose interest over the course of several months.

Answer: "O Lazy bones! Dost thou think God would have given thee arms and legs, if he had not design'd thou should'st use them?" Sign yourself up for upcoming local races and commit yourself by paying the entry fee. Encourage others to run the race with you and support each other. You don't have to break the course record, just finish. Bring your family with you; it's a very social environment. Every participant is a winner.

Excuse #6: My legs hurt when I run.

Answer: "Little strokes, fell great oaks." Start by walking slowly and try to increase either your distance or your exertion level by 10% per week. You can simply add 5 minutes per run per week. Research and find a reputable orthopaedic surgeon who can help you diagnose your musculoskeletal complaints. Ninety-five percent of all aches and pains resolve with several weeks of an over the counter non-steroidal anti-inflammatory such as Advil or Alleve.

Excuse #7: I'm too busy with my work and family right now to exercise for myself.

Answer: "Tomorrow I'll reform, the fool does say; today itself's too late: the wise did yesterday." Exercise is an insurance policy for your physical and mental well being, present and future health. You must regularly sharpen the saw for it to work efficiently.

Excuse #8: I'm too tired.

Answer: "All things are easy to Industry; all things are difficult to Sloth." Every runner knows the hardest part of running is the decision to run and the first five minutes of the run. Once the initial training period is over, exercise will increase your energy and vitality. Just plan a short walk or run. Once you get started you will get stronger and you will feel better.

Excuse#9: Running makes me eat more.

Answer: Drink plenty of water after you run and read Chapter 4.

Excuse #10: I don't want to join a gym, it's too expensive.

Answer: Walking and running are free.

<u>**Take Home Points:**</u>

1. **Exercise one hour a day**

2. **Exercise is a lifelong activity**

3. **Walking is good for you**

4. **Benefits of exercise far outweigh the costs**

7

Motivation

What is going to get you started, keep you going when it's dark and cold? How will you go on when you are alone? What is going to help you rebound from your inevitable setback? Don't fall into the lapse, relapse, and final collapse trap. Recognize when it finally happens to you (and it will) and get back on track. When it comes to motivation, one must keep in mind the Oracle of Delphi's inscription "Know Thyself." One critical key to successful behavioral programs is that each person is an individual and that each person must find what works within the confines of their personality and environment. Motivation must come from many areas including social support, social networks, personal goal commitment and consistency[38], finding a mentor, contingency contracts and personal values.

Success begins in the home. Your wife/husband/significant other must be on board and willing to actively support you and encourage your efforts wholeheartedly. You must discuss your entire plan for getting in shape, soup to nuts, beginning to end. Discuss the history, reasoning, methods and, most importantly, goals. Ask this person to solemnly promise to ignore cries for another piece of cake, ice cream run, or third helping of mashed potatoes. There will be an extinction burst at some point and you will be tortured by the Siren's call from the cookie jar. Your significant other must aggressively encourage your exercise. Your family[39] must be instructed to plug their ears like the crew of Odysseus to ignore your cries to jump ship:

> From Circe Odysseus had learned that they must pass the island of the Sirens. These were marvelous singers whose voices would make a man forget all else, and at last their song would steal his life away. Moldering skeletons of those they had lured to their death lay banked high up around them where they sat singing on the shore. Odysseus told his men about them and that the only way to pass them safely was for each man to stop his ears with wax. He himself, however, was determined to hear them, and he proposed that the crew should tie him to the mast so strongly that he could not get away

40

however much he tried. This they did and drew near the island, all except Odysseus deaf to the enchanting song. He heard it and the words were even more enticing than the melody, at least to a Greek. They would give knowledge to each man who came to them, they said, ripe wisdom and a quickening of the spirit. "We know all things which shall be hereafter upon the earth." So rang their song in the lovely cadences, and Odysseus' heart ached with longing. But the ropes held him and that danger was safely passed.

Your workplace must also adjust to the new program. Certain self-imposed restrictions at work are mandatory. There is to be no junk food readily available to you. You can't keep fire and gasoline together. At this very moment 20 feet away from me sits a box of chocolates and candies a patient of ours brought to our office to thank us for taking care of him. I was offered to take some. Everyone in the office laughed at me because they knew I wouldn't eat any of it. I then picked up every packet of candy and read the calorie content of each piece of candy. One of the bags of chocolate covered peanuts contained 1,600 calories! I could snarf that down before I finished reading my daily emails. One by one I read the calories and looked at everyone in the office. I made sure I got eye contact. After I read the calorie counts to the entire staff, a hush permeated the room.

Make It Work

You must be able to exercise for an hour within your daily schedule. Either start your day later or end it earlier. If your income decreases slightly, so be it. You must avoid lunch partners who tend to overeat, eat too fast, or who have inappropriate eating behaviors discussed in Chapter 3. When you are thinking about relapsing into old behaviors don't be unnecessarily influenced by the wrong people. Either eat alone or surround yourself with light, slow eaters. A period of active weight loss can be a period of personal weakness and vulnerability. Robert Cialdini's book on Influence[38] describes these mechanisms clearly:

> In general, when we are unsure of ourselves, when the situation is unclear or ambiguous, when uncertainty reigns, we are most likely to look to and accept the actions of others as correct.

Establish new social exercise and diet networks. Find an exercise partner who fits with your personality, time schedule, and physical capacity. It may take some time and searching. Pairing up with a running partner forces you to get out of bed and meet him or her. It takes the wind out of the little devil who in the morning suggests hitting the snooze button to get another hour of sleep. Develop several partners and alternate them for variety. Find people who exercise slower than your pace, the same as your pace, and faster than your pace. Be creative in your exercise pattern. On some days I time my runs to connect with more than one person at different locations. It forces us to exercise at an exact time and be at exact locations. Spend time on it like you would a project at work, it's important. Running groups training for a marathon can be found in every city. Seek these exercise groups and join them. They will influence you to continue your positive behaviors.

Set personal goals. Write them down and describe them in detail to the important people in your life. I suggest an exercise goal in the future like a certain distance race and preferably a BMI of 24.9. Be focused on your commitment and your goal. Setting a goal in public with your friends and family will force you to stay consistent with your statement and meet your goal. As Robert Cialdini describes:[38]

> Like the other weapons of influence, this one (consistency) lies deep within us, directing our actions with quiet power. It is quite simply, our desire to be (and to appear) consistent with what we have already done. Once we make a choice or take a stand, we will encounter personal and interpersonal pressures to behave consistently with that commitment...a high degree of consistency is normally associated with personal and intellectual strength. It is the heart of logic, rationality, stability, and honesty...commitments should be active, public, effortful, and freely chosen (uncoerced)...something special happens when people put their commitments on paper: They live up to what they have written down.

Contingency Contracts

Make a contingency contract with yourself and others. A simple and easy contingency contract is signing up with a friend or group to run a race. There will be a small entry fee involved. If you do not run the race you will feel the pain of the wasted money. Your exercise partners will encourage you to complete the race and you will have a goal for your training regimen. Lastly, you will want to avoid the embarrassment of not running the race after publicly informing everyone of your intent to do so. You will strive to be consistent. After you run one race, sign up for another, then another. If you choose not to run, sign up to swim, bicycle, play a sport, or even walk.

Make more than one contingency contract. A deposit-refund system[40] minimizes dropout rates in weight reduction programs to less than 10%. One example is obtaining a cashiers check and giving it to a trusted friend who is disciplined and strong willed. This "executor" friend must then be instructed to implement an agreement in a certain time period. Unless you meet your exercise or weight goal in the certain time period, the check is to be sent to a selected charity. Some people suggest that the charity should be for a cause you feel strongly about, either against or for. If you meet the goal the check is returned to you. Write a one paragraph contract and both of you sign it. The friend is to ignore any pitiful cries of remorse if you do not meet your goal.

A smaller and simpler contingency contract is one that I use with my running partner Charles. I picked him for the contract because when it comes to running, he is a 145 pound Sherman Tank. Initially I was thinking of hiring a trainer. There is some inducement to stay compliant if you do not follow up with your sessions, but one could easily count the money as a sunk cost once it's out of your hands. A better strategy is to write a simple contract with a running partner and friend for a certain period of time. You give the running partner a small sum of money, in my case $20. If you ever back out of a running rendezvous you lose the $20 and you have to give him another $20. This small inducement has motivated me to never back out of a running date. The humiliation of Charles taking my twenty dollars for doing nothing is incentive enough to comply with the running schedule.

The fact is people value loss more than they do gain, even if the loss and gain are the same amount. For example, people give a higher value to the loss of $1,000 dollars than they would an equivalent gain of $1,000 dollars, all things being equal. Daniel Kahneman received the Nobel Prize in Economics in 2002 for the "Prospect Theory[41]" that describes this human behavior.

Initially I made a contract with myself to reward myself for reaching a goal of weight loss or exercise endurance. It didn't motivate me a bit. What did motivate was a contract where I would lose money if I didn't meet a goal. Why not use Daniel Kahneman's economic findings to help you with your goals?

Find a running mentor to help you. Find one or more people who have attained your set goals in the past and who have maintained them. The best mentors are true partners and should meet Warren Buffet's criterion of someone you admire, trust and respect. Exercise with them and talk about your training regimen. This will be one more person you would not want to disappoint by failing to meet your goals.

Handling Pain

While you consistently exercise you will incur one or more injuries or painful conditions. These pains will come and they are to be expected "…for man is born for trouble, as sparks fly upward…[42]." Exercise-induced injuries are not barriers but small hurdles in your way. The question is, do you run into the barrier and fall head first and fail, or do you run over it or around it? In orthopaedic practice, I've encountered two ends of the spectrum when it comes to people's ability to deal with painful conditions, I call them Sensitive Sally and Silent Sal. Both are real people with real problems.

Sensitive Sally was a 24-year-old woman whose chief complaint was coccydynia, or pain along the area of the "tailbone." When I came into the room she was sitting quietly on the exam table. Every 10 to 15 seconds she would shift her weight a little in a fidgety manner to avoid a painful position. When she shifted you could hear a small mouse-like groan. Her younger well-coifed sister sat in a chair next to her. The sister's stiffly prepared hair rose well above and beyond a six inch radius from her head and was accented on the top with a bright pink bow. If the sister were drawn by an artist, she would easily fit as a background character of any Dr. Seuss book. Sensitive Sally in contrast was thin, conservatively well-dressed, and the picture of youthful beauty.

Sensitive Sally quietly explained her history of pain in the tailbone. She had seen many doctors and had followed every treatment regimen. She had taken almost every available non-steroidal anti-inflammatory in the market. She had sat on every protective plastic donut device. No matter what she did, every time she plunked down on the ole keister she had pain in her tailbone. On a table next to her was a stack of films three inches in height of the tests that were taken to workup her condition. Her personal radiographic library included multiple x-rays, MRI's, CT scans, bone scans and bone density studies. When I reviewed them one by one, each had the same diagnosis: normal anatomy. She had already obtained consults from neurological, psychiatric, genecology, and medical experts. She was married, no children, with no other medical problems. Upon reviewing her medications I was flabbergasted at the dose of methadone she was taking—120 milligrams a day!

I was so shocked I put my hand on my forehead. I couldn't believe it. She was on a massive dose of narcotics. I looked at the sister, who said, "You have to know her like I do. She has a VERY high pain tolerance." Her examination revealed no other abnormalities but tenderness along the coccyx or tailbone area. Just lightly touching the skin in the area almost made her jump off the exam table.

There is a procedure of removing the end of the coccyx to help with coccy-dynia, but I felt there was a good probability this patient would never have pain relief despite a technically perfect surgical treatment. She seemed focused on her pain. The pain was a major defining aspect of her life. When she heard there was a chance the surgery might not work she became tearful. I reflexively handed her a Kleenex. The sister began to get angry. While she was crying she mumbled if I could refill her methadone prescription. When I said no, she became furious and they both stormed out of the office. As she passed me by, the sister looked up and gave me a mean glare.

The other end of the spectrum is Silent Sal. Silent Sal was an 80-year-old man with a chief complaint of mild difficulty walking. I had taken care of his wife for many years, and she had recently passed away. He had always been by her side, with all of her difficulties. He was always very supportive. His questions and expectations were always reasonable. Although I had known him for many years by taking care of his wife and his athletic grandsons for their sports injuries, this was the first time I had seen him as a patient. He apologized for coming in for such a trivial problem, and he promised it would be short.

As always he was very nice and smiled frequently. Silent Sal owned a successful business. He worked every day of his life, even though he probably could have retired many years ago. He liked working. I asked him to describe his problem further, and I asked, "Where do you feel the pain?" He put his hand up to stop me like a traffic cop and corrected me by stating, "It's not pain, but rather a stiff-ness in the feet, a mild problem when I walk. I just can't explain it. It's not a very big deal." I asked him if he had ever taken any medicine for the problem and he curtly replied "Never." I asked him if I could take a look at what he was talking about. He took off his shoe and sock to show me his problem.

His feet were terribly deformed from arthritis. The big toe was angled nearly 90 degrees to the rest of his foot. On the joint, there was a terrific abundance of bone spur formation. The x-ray showed terrific joint destruction everywhere from arthritis. While I was looking at the x-ray I asked him again in an incredu-lous tone, "You don't have any pain at all?"

"Not really," he calmly replied. Something didn't make sense. I smelled a rat. After looking at the x-ray I went back to the exam table and decided to test some-thing. I took his big toe and started to move it back and forth to see how much motion he had. He immediately put his hand on mine to stop me and he gri-maced. "Don't do that," he whispered. I stopped immediately as I knew the answer to my question. I gave him a prescription for some inserts for his shoe and he was so happy you would have thought I had cured him entirely on the spot.

Further psychological analysis of these two cases would take hours upon hours and is probably beyond my expertise on many levels. I take the lessons at face value. During exercise there will be some slight mechanical problems that can easily be nursed with common sense treatments of relative rest, decrease or alteration of activity, and simple over-the-counter non-steroidal anti-inflammatory medications like Ibuprofen or Naprosyn. These overuse injuries of activity are hurdles, not impediments.

Get Motivated

Meeting your goals can be a lonely exercise. What motivates you and who are you?

> When Hercules[39] was a young man, two maidens came to him. Arête represented virtue; Kakia was vice. Kakia offered Hercules pleasure and riches if he would follow her. Arête offered him only glory for a lifelong struggle against evil. Hercules chose to be guided by Arête.

Motivation varies among individuals. Each person must set their goals and reach them through their own personal inspiration. Find the motive that drives you and then focus on the goal at all times. There is no way to achieve anything of value without first setting the goal and then focusing.

Be disciplined. Discipline is the basis of success and greatness. As described by Edith Hamilton[43],

> What constitutes Rome's greatness, in the last analysis, is that powerful as these were in her people there was something still more powerful; ingrained in them was the idea of discipline, the soldier's fundamental idea.

8

Final Thoughts

Once the final weight goals have been met, what are the results? Is life better? Can you keep the weight off for years? Do you look great in clothes? Is the return address on your stationery Shangri-La? Are you sitting alone in your basement in silence with your legs crossed, humming the hot sauce diet mantra while experiencing Nirvana?

I can say some things with certainty. None of my previous clothes fit. Although my shirts are still fine, all of my pants are really baggy. I look terrible in clothes now because I'm way too cheap to buy anything new. Some people ask me if I've been sick, or if I've been diagnosed with cancer. Many have a look of gravity and fear when they say it. They're probably afraid that whatever it is, it could be contagious. I'm too superstitious to buy new clothes. It'll be the kiss of death—blow a bunch of money on clothes and the weight will come back on in a couple of days. So I'm stuck looking like Charlie Chaplin, or the lead singer from Talking Heads with my baggy clown-size oversized pants.

Do I get compliments on being thin? Sure, but what good does it do me? The compliments aren't whispered into my ear from a voluptuous Victoria's Secret model. In my case it's from an 80-year-old man chewing a cigar in a clothing store while he's measuring my waist and inseam. All I can think is, "Can you get this over with please?"

If you read any diet books, many state that weight loss vastly improves your sex life. I can't say anything of the sort. My wife has been pregnant or recovering from a C-section and breast feeding the little parasites for the last five years. Our marital relations consist of her poking me in bed with her pointy finger to roll over and stop snoring. I walk a sexual desert wilderness that would make the path of Moses look like a walk down the sands of South Beach Miami. I've resigned myself to the fact that my body's reproductive organs have been mothballed like the great American battleship destroyers of World War II. Sure, they were indispensable and awe-inspiring in their day, and they still are battle ready, but unless another world conflict arises in the distant future, they stay mothballed in the interests of our greater society. There certainly are areas of my body that I can see for the first time in years. That's scary. I used to look like I swallowed a regulation basketball.

Being within normal limits of body weight helps avoid some embarrassing situations where things just didn't fit. Before my weight loss, our family visited the amusement park Cedar Point in Sandusky, Ohio. We waited in line for over an hour to ride the Millennium Force, one of the world's fastest and highest roller coasters. The anticipation was incredible, standing in line watching the coaster flip through loops above our heads. People were screaming at the tops of their lungs.

When we got to the front of the line, one corpulent woman literally could not fit into the cockpit type seats! The staff couldn't let her ride! I felt terrible for her. I broke out into a cold sweat thinking about my own predicament. I have to admit, I just barely fit into it. The teenager who tightened my seat belt had to slam down the restraint with all his might three times for it to fit while I was sucking in my gut. It's a good thing I squeezed into the seat; my cousin, who was next to me, would have never let me hear the end of it. Knowing him he would have laughed about it for years and brought it up every Thanksgiving.

It's the small embarrassing moments that really hurt. Our dining room chairs were subjected to near fatigue failure stress every time I sat in them. I think I've destroyed two of them already. The chair's wooden joints would groan and creak loudly during dinner parties like the deck of a whaling ship. Eating dinner with our family sounded like you were on Captain Ahab's Pequod. You could close your eyes and imagine the boat's wooden planks creaking with every pitch and roll as it chased after the great white whale. In our case it was the white whale, not the ship that was actually making the noise.

I never could cross my legs at the knees. I used to make fun of one of my friends who used to sit this way. I would call him effeminate. The thought didn't cross my mind that my sitting position was not by choice. My thundering thighs kept me from crossing my legs, so I had to put my ankle on my knee. I still think it's effeminate, but I secretly enjoy sitting this way now. I like to show off to myself.

Do I feel great about myself? Of course not! I think I'll always consider myself obese. The sugar cookies on the counter still talk to me, enticing me to eat them. They never stop. If you could get into my head you would think I was schizophrenic from all the voices haunting me to eat more. I'm paranoid that everyone will find out I'm a scrawny fake, just an obese person in disguise.

Yes, there are no more massive rolls of fat. Unfortunately, physical perfection can never be obtained. The massive rolls of fat have been supplanted by excessive rolls of skin. If the skin contracts over time, the eye wanders over to white whiskers, long nose hairs, wrinkles, and countless other imperfections. I do believe that staying thin is good for my self esteem, but I still look middle aged, and every year I look and feel older. It's the price we pay for our existence; we struggle dealing with our mortality. No weight loss or perfect body mass index can fix that problem.

But the daily routine is a lot better right? I think it is. Every day I start out the same. I wake up at 5:00 a.m. At 5:45 a.m. I usually hear my baby daughter start to cry. By that time I have on my running shoes, shorts and reflective vest. I look like someone about to remove litter from the interstate. I bolt out the front door before my wife can ask me to pick up the baby.

Once outside I'm either freezing or too hot. I stretch my joints for one or two minutes in a sort of religious ritual to the musculoskeletal gods. It's my gift to them to protect me from a tendon rupture or strain. I'm convinced it doesn't help anything but I'm too superstitious to stop doing it.

My morning run or exercise regimen is usually an hour long. Is it boring? Rarely. Music and headphones helps pass the time. Is it painful? Yes, but usually only the first 10 to 15 minutes. How do you deal with it? Just barely sometimes, but the longer I continue to run the easier it is. I always remember that if it doesn't feel right after the warm up period, I can always walk home. That happens about 1% of the time.

City Characters

There are people milling about the streets of Baltimore City at that ungodly hour before sunrise. There is the occasional fellow runner. I always do my best to smile and say good morning. Heaven knows what I look like. The serious runners scoff or just plain flat out ignore me. Most of the women runners don't even look at me. Who are these people? I don't know any of them, but it doesn't keep me from giving each and every one of them a nickname and an imaginary life story.

First there's "Hori-Smile." Hori-smile is an approximately 55-year-old man that I encounter at mile four out of six every morning. He's a very punctual and devoted brisk walker. He doesn't do the hilarious flat out power walk, but he's close. I do respect him for exercising. He is 6'0" maybe 210 pounds with a receding hairline and closely cropped white hair. He wears big bulky ear phones and his book-sized cassette tape player is firmly attached to his belt. He obviously hasn't accepted the MP3 iPod digital revolution just yet.

For months Hori-smile ignored my morning salutations. I continued my "Good Morning" assaults in my devotion to an iron discipline of morning social graces. He finally broke down and responded by lifting the lips below his white fluffy caterpillar mustache from an inverted scowl to the horizontal flat position, hence his name: Mr. Hori(zontal)-Smile. I envision him a busy downtown attorney with little time for superficial pleasantries. He's too busy nailing judgments and reviewing affidavits. I'm sure his time is significantly more important than mine, and therefore he never wastes a word by uttering a hello or good morning. His mind probably is constantly ironing out testimony, facts and figures, and important court strategy.

Early in my run I encounter "Gramps on Wheels." Gramps is a 65-year-old bicycle rider who I encounter at mile three out of six. He's never responded to greetings, but I'm convinced he can't hear anything. He's thin and very gray. He wears a stylish black helmet and official skin-tight cycling attire. He sports a large gray Santa Claus type beard. The beard is frayed and wind-worn from the shear velocity of his pedaling. I assume his hearing aid is turned off to avoid petty distractions like a voice or an oncoming city bus horn. He appears to be in excellent physical shape. I picture him a Hopkins physics professor, getting in his exercise just before his daily lecture on differential equations. He can't be bothered by social graces as he ponders the mysteries of the physical universe.

Along the way are many other characters. There's the homeless man who sleeps in the bus stop shelter. I always assumed he was an old man in an overcoat waiting for his bus downtown to go to work, resting his eyes. It wasn't until one day when I doubled my six mile loop to cover 12 miles that I saw him slumped over in exactly the same position one hour later.

I do feel better being thinner. I still hear my joints pop and crack in the morning as I walk down the steps to get the morning paper. I'm constantly hungry. I don't think that will ever change as long as I live.

One thing is for sure, the specter of overeating still haunts me everyday. But now I can laugh at him.

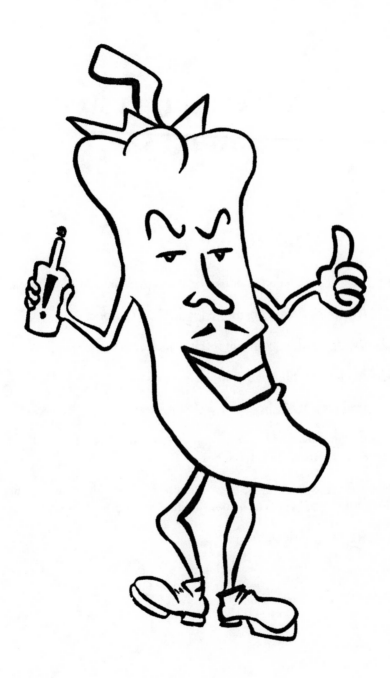

9

Top Ten Suggested Snacks

1. **Push Back:** A teaspoon of hot sauce in a cup of tomato juice. Calories: 60

2. **Golden Greek Pepperoncini Peppers** (HOT): calories 0

3. **Giardiniera/Pickled vegetables** (HOT): calories 0

4. **Pickles, kosher dill small**: calories, 5 per pickle

5. **Mustard for sandwiches**: calories, 0-5 per teaspoon

6. **Fruit**: One apple, banana, orange, pear, one cup of strawberries, blueberries, grapes, or cherries: 70-100 calories

7. **100-calorie vegetable servings**: 2 cups of carrots, three cups of broccoli, three cups of bell peppers, 4 cups cauliflower, 30 cherry tomatoes

8. **Lettuce**: one calorie per leaf

9. **Spinach**: one cup raw is 7 calories, two cups frozen boiled is 120 calories

10. **Celery**: one 12-inch stalk is 10 calories

10

Checklist for Success

X Make a personal commitment that you will fulfill each of the following items

Have a discussion with your significant other/family/co-workers about changing the food and drink environment to avoid overeating/excessive calorie intake. Ask for their support.

Remove all high-calorie beverages from your home and work environment i.e. sodas, and juices. When in doubt, throw it out.

Insert low-calorie beverages into home and work environment within easy access, i.e. water, diet drinks, and diet soda.

Remove all high-calorie foods and snacks from your home and work environment, i.e. chips, cookies, candies, and cake. When in doubt, throw it out.

Insert low-calorie food and snacks into your home and work environment, i.e. see Chapter 9.

Write down the environments and situations where your eating behaviors are abnormal. Create a plan to avoid them.

Create your own personal athletic goals/endeavors to be reached in 1 month, 3 months and 6 months, i.e. be able to run five miles, swim 10 laps, bike for an hour, or walk 10 miles.

Search for and find at least one exercise partner on your block or within a very short distance from your home.

Search for and find at least one exercise partner from your work environment.

Search for and find at least one exercise partner from your social circle.

Find an exercise group that meets regularly once a week, i.e. running club, bicycling club, walking club OR sign up for a regular once a week exercise class.

Sign up for a race/competition/exercise fund raiser and influence your exercise partners to join you (i.e. www.active.com has a large selection).

Buy a dependable scale for your bathroom and measure yourself first thing in the morning to keep track of your weight.

Buy an inexpensive kitchen scale to measure the weight of the food you eat so that you can calculate calories.

Buy a small calorie reference book to monitor your calories and understand what you eat. You can also use a website, i.e. www.nutritiondata.com, www.calorie-count.com, or www.thecaloriecounter.com.

Buy several bottles of hot sauce for your home and work environment.

Buy hot peppers from the grocery store for blow-outs.

Buy a 22 inch x 28 inch piece of poster board to make an exercise calendar/chart to insert your daily exercise accomplishments, caloric intake, and weight. Insert your races and goals on the same calendar. Tape the calendar up for easy access in your kitchen or hallway. Update the chart daily.

Change your work schedule start time to accommodate morning exercise.

Buy a pair of comfortable running/walking shoes.

Buy an inexpensive stopwatch to monitor both your exercise and the time it takes you to eat your meals.

Buy a pair of portable headphones/music player/MP3/iPod if music helps you exercise. Keep the music current and fun.

Sit down with your significant other and thoroughly explain your problem, your goals, and your diet restrictions and seek their full support. This is probably the most important requirement for success.

Create a stock answer and excuse to avoid high-calorie meal environments, i.e. working dinners.

Create a long-term contingency contract with an executor regarding your long-term weight goal, i.e. $100 dollars to be donated to a charity on a certain date if a certain weight is not achieved. Make the details clear on the contract with regards to timing and the scale to be used.

Create a short-term contingency contract with an executor and exercise partner, i.e. if you do not show up for exercise you will pay $10 to be donated to charity. There can be no exceptions or excuses.

Find an exercise mentor who has experience in your chosen exercise method to discuss issues, setbacks, plans, goals, etc.

Discuss your weight-loss plans with your physicians and order necessary tests, i.e. cholesterol, stress test, etc.

Find a local orthopaedic surgeon/physiatrist for an injury assessment if it occurs.

Take a before photograph for your records.

Buy tomato juice or your favorite soup for a "pushback."

Buy/borrow a book on your favorite/chosen exercise to understand it.

Buy a bottle of an anti-inflammatory medicine for minor aches and pains. Make sure this is safe for you by consulting with your doctor.

About the Author

Spiro Antoniades was born and raised in Prince Georges County, Maryland, a suburb of Washington D.C. He earned the degrees of Bachelor of Arts and Medical Doctorate at the John Hopkins University School of Medicine. After completing an orthopaedic surgical residency at Union Memorial Hospital in Baltimore, Maryland, he acquired further spinal surgery fellowship training in Chicago, Illinois at Rush University Medical Center and Shriners Hospital for Children. His knowledge on exercise and nutrition has been based from medical school, post-graduate training, medical practice, and reading on his own in the library. He currently lives in Baltimore City with his wife and three children, where he also actively practices orthopaedic surgery.

Endnotes

1. Gardner, Martin. The Annotated Alice-the definitive edition. 2000.W.W.Norton & C Ltd

2. http://www.cdc.gov/nccdphp/dnpa/bmi/index.htm

3. Feldman: Sleisenger & Fordtran's Gastrointestinal and Liver Disease 7th Edition 2002

4. Stedman's medical dictionary—25th edition 1990 p.426

5. http://www.cdc.gov/diabetes/pubs/general.htm#impaired

6. http://www.cdc.gov/nccdphp/dnpa/obesity/defining.htm

7. http://www.cdc.gov/nccdphp/dnpa/obesity/trend/maps/index.htm

8. Marcus Aurelius (121-180) Meditations viii.22

9. http://www.mcdonalds.com/app_controller.nutrition.index1.html

10. Simpson J.A., and Weiner, E.S.C. The Oxford English Dictionary second edition Clarendon Press Oxford 1986

11. http://www.health.gov/dietaryguidelines/dga2005/document/

12. http://www.iom.edu/Object.File/Master/21/372/0.pdf

13. Sclafani, A. and Springer D. Dietary Obesity in Adult Rats: Similarities to Hypothalamic and Human Obesity Syndromes. Physiology and Behavior, 1976, 17, pp 461-471

14. McHugh, PR, and Slavney PR. The Perspectives of Psychiatry. Baltimore: Johns Hopkins University Press 1983 and 1998

15. Wedding, Danny. Behavior and Medicine. 1990. Mosby-Year Book, Inc.

16. Skinner, BF The Behavior of organisms: An experimental approach. 1938. Englewood Cliffs, NJ: Prentice Hall

17. Govindarajan VS and Sathyanarayana MN. Capsicum—Production, Technology, Chemistry, and Quality. Part V Impact on Physiology, Phar-

macology, Nutrition, and Metabolism; Structure, Pungency, Pain, and Desensitization Sequences. Crit. Rev. Food Science and Nutrition. 1991; 29(6):435-474 Review

18. Winek CL. Pepper Sauce Toxicity. Drug and Chemical Toxicology, 5(2), 89-113 (1982)

19. http://ptcl.chem.ox.ac.uk/MSDS/glossary/ld50.html

20. Feldman: Sleisenger & Fordtran's Gastrointestinal and Liver Disease 7th Edition 2002

21. Tadataka Yamada 3rd Edition Textbook of Gastroenterology. Chapter 64 Lippincott Williams and Wilkens

22. http://www.healthierus.gov/dietaryguidelines/

23. McArdle, William D. Essentials of exercise physiology. 1994. Lee and Febiger

24. Williams, Melvin. Nutritional Aspects of Human and Physical Athletic Performance. 2nd edition. Charles C. Thomas Publications 1985

25. Bergstrom J et al. Diet, muscle, glycogen, and physical performance. Acta Physiol. Scand., 71:140, 1967

26. Stunkard AJ. Obesity: International Handbook of Behavior Modifications and Therapy

27. L'Abate, L., Farrar, J.E., Serritella, D.A., Handbook of Differential Treatment for Addictions. Allyn and Bacon 1992

28. http://www.cfsan.fda.gov/list.html

29. Brownell, K.D. Obesity: Understanding and Treating a Serious, Prevalent, and Refractory Disorder. J Consulting and Clinical Psychology 1982, Vol 50, No. 6, 820-840

30. http://www.health.gov/dietaryguidelines/dga2005/recommendations.htm

31. http://www.cdc.gov/nccdphp/dnpa/physical/pdf/MSA_2000_walking.pdf

32. http://www.runningusa.org/cgi/mar_repts.pl

33. Covey, SR. The Seven Habits of Highly Effective People. Free Press (2004)p 289

34. http://www.exrx.net/Aerobic/WalkCalExp.html

35. Fixx, James. The Complete Book of Running. Random House NY 1977

36. Dempsey RL, Incidence of sports and recreation related injuries in hospitalizations in Wisconsin in 2000. Inj. Prev 2005; 11: 91-96

37. http://www.neurosurgerytoday.org/what/patient_e/sports.asp

38. Cialdini R.B. Influence Science and Practice fourth edition Allyn and Bacon 2001

39. Hamilton Edith. Mythology. The New American Library, Little Brown and Company, Boston, MA. 17ᵗʰ printing 1962

40. Hagan RL. The drop-out problem: Reducing attrition in obesity research. Behavior Therapy 1976,7,463-471

41. Kahneman, Daniel, and Amos Tversky (1979) "Prospect Theory: An Analysis of Decision under Risk", Econometrica, XVLII (1979), 263-291.

42. Job 5:7

43. Hamilton, Edith. The Roman Way. W.W.Norton & Company Inc. NY 1932

978-0-595-41187-0
0-595-41187-8

Printed in the United States
65096LVS00005B/442